THE CHIROPRACTIC HANDBOOK FOR PATIENTS

DIRK TOUSLEY

Third Edition

A WHITE DOVE BOOK
WHITE DOVE PUBLISHING CO.

THE CHIROPRACTIC HANDBOOK FOR PATIENTS
by Dirk Tousley

Editorial Consultant: David Grayson Lees

Copyright © 1983, 1984, 1985 by
White Dove Publishing Co.

Third edition, expanded 1985
Library of Congress Catalog Card Number: 83-50885

ISBN: 0-914541-01-3

Published by:
WHITE DOVE PUBLISHING CO.
10605 Winner Road
Independence, Missouri 64052
Printed in the United States of America

Nothing can resist an idea whose time has come.
—Victor Hugo

*To my best friend and wife, Jacqueline,
and to my son, Adam.*

ACKNOWLEDGEMENTS

An acknowledgement of everyone who has helped me with this book would include the names of more than 3,000 chiropractors I have served in the past seventeen years as a business consultant.

Without knowing it, each of them taught me the beauty of chiropractic and how meaningful it is to be a chiropractor. In a very real sense, each of them appears in this book.

Also, I am grateful to the American Chiropractic Association for information on chiropractic colleges and the history of Physiological Therapeutics in chiropractic.

And special thanks to Golden Touch Press for permission to quote from two pamphlets I wrote for them several years ago: "The Amazing Story of Chiropractic" and "How Chiropractic Heals." This symbol † appears twice in this book indicating those quotations.

CONTENTS

Truth happens *to be an idea. It becomes true, is made true by events . . . Its verity is in fact an event, a process: the process namely of its verifying itself, its verification. Its validity is the process of its validation.*

—*William James*

Chiropractic . . . and You

In its own time, the mantle of fame has gradually embraced chiropractic. Certainly, chiropractors themselves have not pushed for it. They just show up at the office every morning and get sick people well, often after other doctors have given up.

Although chiropractors frequently accomplish "healing miracles," theirs is usually a workaday world. Primarily using their trained hands in gentle manipulation of the spine they treat a broad spectrum of human miseries from A to Z . . . even including the common cold.*

Characterized in the past as "Old Doc" who will "pop your back when you're all stoved up," times have changed. And if fame is a payoff, the chiropractor should be smiling now.

Chiropractic in the Limelight

Today's chiropractors find themselves in the limelight on the healing arts stage, "in" doctors to a

---

* See "Infectious Diseases" later in this book.

substantial number of people who have discovered that *whole* health obtained through *drugless* chiropractic methods is far superior, more satisfying, longer lasting and much less expensive than drugs and surgery.

They have found that modern chiropractic methods are painless, and since there is no prescription-fill at the drug store on the way home, there are no debilitating side effects or addictions.

Thus, to many people, chiropractic means freedom.

Growing Popularity

The chiropractor's uncomplicated, natural approach to health has brought a burgeoning popularity due mainly to word-of-mouth acclaim by satisfied, enthusiastic patients.

Just last year an estimated 5,000,000 Americans, men, women, and children *switched to chiropractors* for their health problems after hearing some good news about chiropractic from friends, relatives, or business associates.

Yet, ironically, the road to universal acceptance still eludes the chiropractor. Though chiropractors are licensed in all of the fifty states, considered a primary health care provider by the United States Department of Health and Human Services, and their patients' claims are paid by virtually all health insurance companies, there are still millions of people who desperately need a chiropractor—but who are scared off by the medical establishment's vicious and unremitting anti-chiropractic campaign.

This biased attitude by the medical establishment toward chiropractic is not new. They have always felt that they and they alone should have absolute, sole discretion and dominion over *all* health issues and that anyone also treating disease is an interloper into their sacrosanct bailiwick, "their" territory. Smear tactics against chiropractic have never let up since chiropractic was brought forth to the world nearly a century ago.

Certainly chiropractic would have long been sunk except for two factors: chiropractors ignored the attacks as best they could and just kept on getting sick people well. And their patients also ignored the propaganda and just kept on spreading the good word about how chiropractic had helped them.

The big losers, of course, have been the innocent sick—perhaps people like you—brain-washed against the very method that could have helped them.

Fortunately, it is impossible "to fool all of the people all of the time." Even when criticism has been at its worst, the chiropractor's patients have known better. But untold millions who chiropractic could have helped were kept away.

Medical "Wonders"?

But times are changing. History shows us that all despotic propaganda is eventually negated by the truth. The truth is that despite all the "wonders" of medical technology, many of the advances in one area have been offset by regressions in others. For example, while longevity figures have gone up, the quality of those extra years is highly questionable. Thousands upon thousands of "old people" live a half-life in the fog of senility and tranquilizers, warehoused in "old people's homes," an appropriate name

11

regardless of what some call a geriatric facility.

Hospital costs are out of control. And the benign violence of surgery is frequently misplaced, misdirected, misused and overused . . . while drugs have become a "quick fix" that too often leads to a cruel addiction. It is estimated that every night up to thirty million Americans take some kind of drug just to get to sleep.

To be sick has become a way of life. However, some people don't even live long enough to become chronically ill. Of the eighteen most technologically advanced countries, the United States is thirteenth in infant mortality.

Now, that's sick!

Restoring Wholeness

The so called "mainstream" health care system, which views the attainment of health as a battle against disease clearly does not work very well.

Conversely, like the difference between night and day, chiropractors see the attainment of health as a process of maintaining and restoring the innate *wholeness* of each patient.

Introducing you to how they go about it is the purpose of this handbook.

Chiropractic . . . and A Dramatic Discovery

The discovery of chiropractic principles was inevitable. It's easy to see that now, nearly one hundred years after the fact, especially in light of the social context of the late nineteenth century.

As that century went into its last quarter or so, there wasn't much excitement going on, at least compared to its middle years. The wretched Civil War and the bitter Reconstruction period were over. The west was nearly won and there just didn't seem to be much left to do or many more frontiers to conquer. The times were slow paced . . . a horse and buggy world . . . and the mood of the nation was in limbo.

Drama of Discovery

Then, suddenly, like a continuing succession of artillery bursts, there appeared on this placid national scene an astounding variety and number of dramatic scientific and industrial inventions and processes, ideas and concepts which forevermore enhanced the quality of man's life.

13

Chiropractic was one of these.

The sudden burst of activity from a nation that appeared to be asleep is still without adequate explanation. But for whatever reason, it seemed that wherever there was a *need* to be filled during those turn-of-the-century years, someone appeared on the scene to fill it.

Edison was one. He saw that people were tired of fumbling around by candlelight, so he invented the electric light.

Bell, another "dreamer," made it possible for people to "reach out and touch someone."

Roentgen invented the X-ray.

And on and on. One after another and in clusters, forward-looking people came forward with thousands of "brand new" devices, items, processes and services and presented them to a public hungry for change.

Then, a peculiar thing happened. As people began to see that change was possible, virtually every aspect of living that was uncomfortable or didn't work well was put up for examination and possible change.

The practice of medicine was no exception.

In those days, patent medicines were rampant and largely ineffective. The medical profession was attempting to organize itself, establish standards of competency and eliminate quackery within its own ranks—striving to become scientific and thereby discover more of the causes of human disease. Here, in the health sciences, there was an enormous need to be filled. It was Daniel David Palmer's fate to fill it.

Dr. Palmer's Breakthrough

Working alone, like so many successful "backyard

scientists" of the time, Palmer discovered the principles of chiropractic through his own research and genius. Here's the story of how it all began:

It was September 18, 1895, and Dr. Palmer was in his office in Davenport, Iowa, carrying on a shouted conversation with the nearly deaf janitor of the building, Harvey Lillard.

Lillard was explaining in shouts to Palmer that about 17 years before while working in a cramped, stooped position, something had "popped" in his back. Since that time, his hearing had become progressively worse.

Dr. Palmer, a curious, intelligent man, examined Lillard's back and found a painful, misaligned vertebra at the spot where something had "popped" 17 years before. He suspected a connection between this misaligned vertebra and Lillard's impaired hearing . . . and reasoned that if something had gone wrong in the man's back to cause deafness, the correction of the misaligned vertebra should bring back Lillard's hearing.

Using his hands, Palmer repositioned the vertebra with a gentle thrust. Lillard's hearing improved immediately. In that moment, Palmer made the breakthrough that had eluded the greatest medical minds of all the ages . . . he had discovered a major cause of human suffering and disease.

During the next few days, Palmer continued the "hand treatments" of Lillard's spine. Within a week, Lillard was able to hear as well as anybody; he told everybody who would listen about Dr. Palmer's "hand treatments." Palmer named the science "chiropractic" after two Greek works *cheir* and *praktikis*, which translates into "done by hand."

Dr. Palmer's fame spread quickly as he continued to prove that his hand treatments were effective in many different diseases and conditions. Soon, ailing people were traveling from near and far to receive the treatments from Dr. Palmer.

Founding the Palmer School

Realizing he alone would be unable to give his new-found knowledge broad outlet, he founded the Palmer School of Chiropractic in Davenport. †

While many of Palmer's first students were medical doctors, the medical establishment soon repudiated chiropractic and its philosophy and theories, dubbing them "unscientific quackery." They maintained that while Palmer's theory might explain positive results in some conditions, his explanation of Lillard's cure contained a fundamental error. They contended that Lillard's miraculous recovery was only coincidental, rather than consequential to Palmer's treatment. They maintained there was no known nerve connection between the treated vertebra and the nerves involved in hearing. This early criticism was to haunt chiropractors for many years.

Since then, many medical, osteopathic and chiropractic physicians have reported similar instances of restoration of hearing following spinal manipulation. Such reports are sufficient in number to remove the possibility of coincidence.

Today, neurologists are still unable to trace the *direct nerve circuits* involved, but readily admit the complexity of the nervous system with its plexuses, ganglions, and billions of internuncial connections could easily accommodate several explanations of how Lillard's hearing was restored.

Although the exact mechanism of Lillard's case is still unknown, results speak for themselves.

Medical physicians, too, utilize methods and treatments that unquestionably work, but whose mechanisms are not fully understood. For instance, the explanation of how general anesthesia works has many theories, but none of them have been scientifically proven. Yet, anesthesia is used thousands of times every day because it works—though no one knows exactly how or why.

Working with "What Works"

No doubt, someday, such questions concerning both medical and chiropractic science will be answered. In the meantime, we have to work with . . . what works.

Today, from the humble beginning of just one doctor and just one patient, many fine chiropractic colleges are found throughout the United States, Canada and the world, currently filled by more than 10,000 enthusiastic, dedicated students.

Dr. Palmer's premise is accepted, and legally recognized in all of the 50 states, the Canadian provinces and many foreign countries. Chiropractic is the largest of the "non-medical" healing professions. Palmer's science, the product of a man who refused to be beaten down by prejudice, superstition or ignorance, is practiced throughout the world because it gets sick people well.

Chiropractic . . . and Wholeness

The words "whole" and "health" have a common origin in the Old English word *hal*. Centuries ago, "whole" was spelled *hal*. It meant "health." So to be healthy was to be whole.

Today, when you greet a friend by asking, "How are you? How's your health?" it's just the modern mode of inquiring "Are you whole?" . . . an abbreviated message that asks, "Are the structure and function of your body integrated and compensating for this moment's environment? Is your body balanced to the pull of gravity? Are your heart, lungs, other organs and systems coordinated and integrated in response to directions from your nervous system?"

"Do you *feel* healthy, *whole?*"

Compared to the ideal structure of the human body as shown and described by the diagrams in a textbook such as *Gray's Anatomy*, you are probably not whole . . . *not* perfectly integrated. But hardly anyone matches that textbook perfection.

When we sum up all of the unhealthful factors we subject our bodies to, it's no wonder we aren't whole.

18

Genetic makeup accounts for some of the discrepancy. Each of us is born stronger or weaker in certain body systems and organs than in others. And as we move through life, some of us don't take very good care of ourselves.

Too, most of us have mental and physical stresses associated with our work and personal lives that tear away at our health, our *wholeness*.

Other hostile forces nip at our health, such as inclement weather, polluted air, adulterated and junk food, impure water, cigarettes, booze, drugs, too much coffee and all the rest of the bio-negative elements making up our culture.

Integrated Structure and Function

Still, regardless of adverse genetic and environmental conditions, we can enjoy health if we don't let our bodies stray too far from *integrated structure and function*.

Sometimes it is said that health is the absence of disease. But, that definition is much too black and white for application to everyday living. A more helpful concept is to visualize health and disease as two *momentums* headed in opposite directions. Disease is the momentum resulting from *dis*integration of the structures and functions of your body. Health is a momentum resulting from *integration* of the structures and functions of your body.

An ageing horse put out to pasture is a prime example of disease momentum prompted by the *dis*integration of the horse's structure and function. Due to his ageing structure, his functions are altered, and that, in turn, alters his structure which, again, alters his function more so . . . an ever-quickening cycle of disintegration accelerating the disease momentum. Obviously, this horse is headed for the glue factory.

Now, let's imagine a thoroughbred pounding down the home stretch with the smell of victory in his nostrils. He demonstrates integrated structure and function as a health momentum. He'll be acknowledged with a garland of roses in the Winner's Circle.

The basic difference between the two horses is that one is disintegrating, *falling apart* in a disease momentum; while the other is still integrated, *whole*, in a health momentum.

The Human Space Suit

The same structure/function principle applies to the human body. It's just that we are so used to thinking of our bodies as a collection of unrelated parts that the wholeness concept may be difficult to understand at first. Perhaps the *space suit analogy* may help.

Your body can be compared to a space suit loaded with integrated electrical, chemical and mechanical apparatus . . . a space suit taking a walk through the earth's environment of changing weather, stress, heavy traffic and all of the other bio-negative forces we just mentioned. *It is a space suit whose mechanism for survival compensates for and matches the ordinary stresses of the earth's environment.*

This space suit is soft and flexible, yet tough and resilient. It has the capacity to think for itself, reproduce and enjoy the fruits of the planet while at the same time coping with its hostility. Most important, the suit has the ability to maintain its own internal environment. What's more, except in extreme circumstances, if its stability is upset it can produce its own cures and oversee its own recuperation. Its material needs are few: food, clothing and shelter.

It sounds almost human, doesn't it?

Like a space suit, the human body is one whole structure, too, made up of billions of cells. Microscopic in size, some cells are long and stringy while others are brick-shaped, flat or irregular, according to the job they have to do.

Similarly-shaped cells group to form the tissues which compose the body's organs. Certain organs work together in a system such as the circulatory system which includes the heart, blood vessels, lymphatic vessels, lymph nodes and spleen.

In total there are nine major systems of the body: skeletal, muscular, endocrine (glands), circulatory, digestive, respiratory, urinary, reproductive and nervous. Each of the systems has been structurally and functionally identified so that we know where each system begins and ends.

But, each system interacts with and thereby affects all the other systems which are in turn interdependent, interrelated and integrated. When we're healthy, they work together to make us *feel whole.*

The "Chord" of Health

Another way to grasp the wholeness concept is to compare it to a chord of music. We know the individual notes are there, but they have merged their identities—all we hear is the chord. In man, the "chord" occurs when each of the body systems blends its structural and functional identity to make up only one structure and function: an integrated, healthy human being, the whole person.

21

But unfortunately, our preoccupation with the conquest of disease is costing us our health . . . our wholeness. We marshall our technological forces to combat a disease uprising in one area of the body, only to have the same or different condition erupt again, perhaps in another area . . . again . . . and again.

The main result has been an ever-widening search for specific potions and drugs to cure specific diseases. Our past is littered with quests for elixirs, ungents, even incantations to cure the human body of this or that.

Each generation of disease healers, in whatever form they present themselves, are sure they have the answers.

Witch doctors prescribed, perhaps, the residue of an owl's foot boiled for five days in the urine of a pregnant goat, or some other bizarre concoction. Today's medical doctor can prescribe thousands upon thousands of manufactured chemical mixtures and compounds designed for specific diseases, pains and conditions in the hope that something from the outside will give us health on the inside.

And such "cures" are often worse than the original disease. Today it is estimated that up to 50% of all hospital admissions are for three major conditions:

(1) iatrogenic—doctor induced or created
(2) pharmacogenic—drug related
(3) nosocomial—hospital related

The terrifying truth is that in many instances, doctors, drugs and hospitals are creating nearly as many diseases as they are curing, and killing some people while they save others.

While there are many benefits of high technology

in health care, we must be continually aware that they carry a high price tag, not only in time and money, but in potentially adverse consequences . . . and therefore should be prescribed very judiciously.

Tunnel Vision

Such high-tech emphasis is tunnel vision with a vengeance, a continual peering into laboratory microscopes in *a search for yet another cure* while almost totally ignoring the body's inherent powers of healing and its more natural means of stimulating and restoring its awesome ability to take care of its own ills.

Indeed, if it weren't for the innate powers of the human body to maintain a desirable internal environment, the human race would never have survived. None of us would be here. Yet, the human race has survived and multiplied for about 500,000 years without benefit of doctoring as we know it today. So, *something* must be working for us. That "something" is the body's innate healing powers and its inclination to be healthy.

Your Body's Environment

The degree of your body's ability to take care of itself depends upon the degree of integration of the body's systems and organs. This concept of integration is not dissimilar to the "ecosystem" of the earth.

We are reminded repeatedly that man's pollution of the air, land, streams and oceans is chipping away at the integration of all the natural systems that make the earth a beautiful place to live.

It is even said that if we don't change our polluting ways quickly, the health of the earth may go past the point of no return. That is, we may overwhelm the ecosystem balance so much that the earth will not be able to bounce back to its old smiling self.

The same principle applies to our own health. It's imperative that all our systems be integrated with each other to make us whole.

Chiropractors concern themselves with the integration of all the body systems through helping to maintain the proper functioning of the nervous system . . . the master system which directly and indirectly controls all the other systems.

Let's take a look at how it works . . .

Chiropractic . . . and The Role of Nerves in Wholeness

There was a time when the nervous system was seen as being a lot like a telephone system. The brain was depicted as the central switchboard, the spinal cord was shown as a trunk line branching out to various "telephones" in the body's parts. That early picture was quite graphic—but highly oversimplified.

Actually, distribution of nerves throughout the body is so intimate and extensive that if we could dissolve away all other tissues, we would still see the form and proportions of the body in gossamer, a phantom body made up entirely of nerves. †

By means of nerve impulses, (electrochemical processes) the nervous system unifies, integrates, controls and directs the functions of your body in the all-important work of achieving its primary goals: survival, wholeness, health, well-being. Even the circulatory and glandular systems—potent directors, controllers, and unifiers themselves—are largely subject to the commands of the nervous system.

Unlike a relatively simple telephone system connecting one location to another, the nervous system's complex "connections" are currently beyond our comprehension. We can grasp only a little of this complexity at a time.

Amazing Complexity

For example, at any given moment, thousands of bits of "information" from just sight and sound alone enter your nervous system and *must be analyzed instantly* to determine your body's appropriate response.

About 99 percent is discarded as unimportant at the moment. While all this is going on, all the other senses are active, too, bombarding the nervous system, demanding answers.

At the same time, the body's many organ and system functions must be tirelessly monitored, directed and unified. Since we can't possibly keep track of all these activities, let's keep it simple to get some idea of the enormity and complexity of the nervous system's responsibilities.

We have already seen that the body is made up of nine major systems (skeletal, muscular, endocrine, circulatory, digestive, respiratory, urinary, reproductive and nervous) each with its own complement of organs and glands, each of whose functions are multifaceted. For example, the pituitary gland secretes at least 150 hormones, and the liver, as another example, has hundreds of known processes.

With this rudimentary example of the number of functions within the body, we see that just the *known* functions of the body's sytems, organs and glands are infinite in their number of actions, reactions and interactions. Enough zeros simply do not exist to represent the totality of the nervous system's scope.

Exquisite Timing

The nervous system must also incorporate exquisite timing. Merely dashing out-of-doors in your bathrobe and pajamas on a snowy morning to get the newspaper instantly calls into play body responses to help you retain body heat, keep from slipping on the snow, find the newspaper in a snowdrift, and at the same time say "hi" to a passing neighbor. The body functions directed and integrated by the nervous system in that little episode involve more computations, permutations, directions and actions than the most sophisticated computer could ever track. And these processes go on and on in every moment of your life, for all of your life. There's no shutting everything down for lunch. As soon as you pick up the newspaper and return to the house, an entire new complex of integrated nerve impulses begin anew.

Just imagine what would happen if you had to stop to think about each of these actions of the nervous system in your daily life.

Fortunately, we only have to pay conscious attention to a tiny fraction of what the nervous system does to keep us whole. When nerve impulses flow smoothly and unimpeded, we enjoy health . . . wholeness.

But, as we shall see, whenever there is interference with normal nerve function, problems are sure to follow.

27

Chiropractic . . .
and How "Pinched"
Nerves Cause Disease

Some people are still skeptical of chiropractic because they are unable to see how a problem in the back could possibly have anything to do with disease inside the body.

Everyone accepts that "pinched" nerves from a "broken" neck can cause complete paralysis of the arms and legs, but many people are unaware that nerves irritated by misaligned vertebrae can also cause dysfunction of the internal organs and systems.

This attitude is typified by the following incident: several years ago the writer was standing in line with a chiropractor at an airport ticket counter. A woman directly in front of the chiropractor was wheezing and coughing with a rather severe asthma attack. The chiropractor said to her, "You really ought to consider seeing a chiropractor for that asthma condition."

Between wheezes, the woman gasped, "Oh, Heavens, no! I don't believe in chiropractors. My doctor told me to stay away from them."

"Well," said the chiropractor (politely), "it's a free country. I guess you can keep your doctor and your asthma as long as you want to."

The woman's attitude about chiropractic would be

funny if it weren't so tragic. The medical profession has been preoccupied with the *drama* of surgery, germs, viruses and infections, and remarkable progress has been made in those areas. But still, 15,000,000 Americans suffer from chronic headaches. Another 28,000,000 have arthritis. Heart disease is still the No. 1 killer in America. Chronic fatigue, high blood pressure and stomach ulcers tarnish the happiness of millions. Hay fever, asthma, sinusitis and emphysema make hundreds of thousands miserable. Neuritis, bursitis and sciatica plague millions more.

Meeting Health Problems Head On

It is the new kind of doctor, the chiropractor, who every day meets these health problems head on. He is the only doctor who recognizes *the cause/effect relationship between pinched nerves in the spine and disease*, both acute and chronic; who sees that the human body can often rid *itself* of pain and disease when interference with normal nerve function is removed through chiropractic adjustments.

A Splendid Design

The design of the spine is indeed most splendid, incorporating flexibility, strength and resilience in its critical role of protecting the spinal cord and nerves. It is also most susceptible to the stresses and strains, knocks and bumps of everyday living and from time to time may require professional help in its maintenance and care. That is the chiropractor's responsibility.

The basis for his philosophy, thought and actions is firmly established, without question, in the anatomy and physiology of the human body. Any definitive textbook on those subjects will show that an adult spine is composed of twenty-four bones called vertebrae. Each vertebra has a hole in its center from top to bottom, and the vertebrae are stacked one on top of another. Like a column of doughnuts, they form a tunnel for the spinal cord.

The vertebrae are held in place by an arrangement of ligaments (connective tissue). A system of muscles attached to the vertebrae can rotate the spine and bend it forward, backwards, and sideways, allowing for a great range of spinal movement while at the same time the vertebrae protect the delicate spinal cord and nerves.

The spinal cord—slightly thicker than a pencil—is suspended from the brain and extends downward through the tunnel formed by the vertebrae. The somewhat smaller major nerve trunks lead from the spinal cord through channels formed by notches in adjacent vertebrae. These notches are called *foramen*.

When these notches are correctly aligned, the nerves leading through them can function properly. If the notches become even slightly misaligned, the channel becomes distorted and the major nerve trunks passing through the channel can become stretched, impinged, entrapped, compressed, pinched or otherwise irritated.

Regardless of the cause, such irritations of the nerve trunk can affect and alter the proper function, sensitivity or conductivity of the nerve and thereby create dysfunction and lowered resistance to infection and disease in the areas or systems of the body served directly or indirectly by that nerve complex.

Chiropractic . . . and Techniques of Treatment

Patients are sometimes curious as to why two different chiropractors might use different techniques for the same condition.

Differences in techniques occur in all the healing professions because doctors usually have several options of approach to the same problem.

For example, all surgeons do not always utilize the same technique in every operation; all medical physicians do not prescribe the same medication for a given condition; and all psychologists do not use identical treatment or counseling techniques.

Chiropractors, too, have many treatment options. For instance, misaligned vertebrae may be corrected in a variety of ways including chiropractic adjustments, manual manipulation, mechanical mobilization, muscle balancing, applied kinesiology, specific reflex techniques, passive motion therapies, manual and motorized traction, along with many other effective techniques.

The selection of techniques to be employed depends upon the nature of the patient's condition and the preference, training, and experience of the individual chiropractor.

Chiropractic . . . and Safety of Treatments

Chiropractic treatments are safe. It is estimated that more than 1,000,000 treatments are received by patients *every day*. Adverse reaction to treatment is very rare.

The safety of chiropractic care is confirmed by the low malpractice insurance premium that chiropractors pay compared to the enormous premiums paid by medical physicians and other health care providers.

This high degree of safety in chiropractic care is primarily due to the thorough examinations that are customarily made preceding treatment. These examinations are designed to screen out conditions for which chiropractic care is not indicated.

Chiropractic . . . and Does it Hurt?

Do chiropractic treatments hurt?

Normally not.

But apprehension that a chiropractic adjustment might be painful sometimes keeps away the very person who needs the treatment the most.

About one million people a day receive chiropractic adjustments. Many have no pain at all when they first come to the chiropractor's office. Some are in mild pain and a few are in severe pain.

If pain is not present in normal movement, the sensation of a chiropractic adjustment is not painful. Instead, there is usually an awareness that something extraordinarily good has just happened.

If pain is already present during normal movement, the pain does not normally increase during the adjusting process and is followed almost always by a *release of pain*.

A common immediate response to a chiropractic adjustment is . . . an audible sigh of relief.

Chiropractic . . . and X-ray

Chiropractic and the X-ray were discovered in the same year, 1895. Chiropractors were among the first doctors to utilize X-ray in their practices; chiropractic research has been instrumental in developing X-ray technology.

X-ray is widely used in the chiropractic profession as a part of the diagnostic procedure, but is never used as a treatment . . . *only for diagnosis.*

Depending on the nature of your complaint, the doctor may make X-ray photographs from different viewpoints. These pictures can help reveal or rule out subluxations, misalignments, distortion of the spinal column, disease of the bone, fractures, malignancy, pelvic imbalance, curvatures and many other conditions that could be present.

The X-ray pictures help the doctor in determining the cause and severity of your problem and what needs to be done to correct it.

Chiropractic . . . and Osteopathic Medicine

The difference between chiropractic and osteopathy is a question that's often asked.

Osteopathy is a system of treatment developed by a medical physician, Dr. Andrew Still, who opened the first College of Osteopathy in 1892.

Dr. Still reasoned that since many health problems are related to impaired circulation, and that many disease processes might also be caused by diminished or reduced circulation of the blood in the affected area, manipulation of the affected disease area would increase the circulation and help the body to restore health.

His manipulation treatments helped many patients, and he proposed his theories and methods to his medical colleagues. But they rejected his theories and therapy. He became the target of attack by the medical hierarchy of that day . . . in much the same way as D.D. Palmer, the discoverer of chiropractic.

Rejected by his own profession, he established the first osteopathic school. In addition to "accepted" medical course work, he instructed students in his theories and methods of manipulation for the purpose of increasing circulation.

Important Distinctions

There are several important distinctions between the original osteopathic philosophies and techniques and chiropractic philosophies and techniques.

Both professions use manipulation as a treatment, but osteopathic manipulations are performed mainly to mobilize tissues and structures for the purpose of stimulating and increasing blood flow into and from the diseased area.

Conversely, chiropractic manipulations, called *adjustments*, are directed primarily to misaligned vertebrae of the spine for the purpose of normalizing the flow of nerve impulses to and from the affected areas.*

Beyond the original philosophical differences of restoring blood supply vs. restoring nerve supply lies the difference in the way the two professions practice today. With few exceptions, most osteopaths function as medical physicians and use very little manipulation. When they do, it is largely in addition to drugs and surgery.

But, *chiropractors use manipulation (chiropractic adjustments) as the primary treatment*. Nutrition and physiological therapeutics are adjunctive and supplemental to the chiropractic adjustments.

---

*Modern osteopathic teachings also recognize the importance of nerve interference.

Because both professions have their roots in manipulative and adjustive methods and have both been the victims of medical propaganda, harrassment and ostracism, chiropractors and osteopaths generally enjoy a harmonious inter-professional relationship and share and refer patients freely.

Chiropractic . . . and Physical Therapy*

Chiropractors are trained extensively in Physiological Therapeutics. As early as 1912, the subject was taught in a chiropractic college and has long been officially recognized as part of chiropractic practice by the American Chiropractic Association.

In addition to manual manipulation of the spine and other joints of the human body, most chiropractors utilize Physiological Therapeutics "modalities" including ultrasound, diathermy, traction, vibratory therapy, electro-muscle stimulation, meridian therapy, acupuncture, acupressure and many others. Such therapeutic measures are utilized in conjunction with and adjunctive to other standard chiropractic techniques and methods. Heat and cold and vapor-coolant sprays for the treatment of "trigger points" are also common procedures.

Helpful Methods

Appropriate modalities are very helpful in acute sprains and strains, and almost essential in obtaining maximum results in chronic conditions affecting the

*See "Scope of Practice" chapter.

38

supporting structures of the vertebrae, muscles, ligaments, fascia and joints. Most vertebral and other joints that have been misaligned for even a short time have developed adhesions, contractures and fixations and the ligaments, muscles and fascia have conformed themselves to the misalignment.

As the chiropractor begins the series of treatments usually required in the gradual realigning of the vertebrae, the associated ligaments and muscles must reshape and reconform themselves, this time to the new realigned position of the vertebrae.

Without supplemental physiological therapeutic treatments, in many cases the rehabilitative process takes a long time. Therapeutic heat and cold, traction, exercise and other physical therapies have proved to be highly effective in speeding up the process.

In some cases, it's possible to get results without these therapies, but there's no question that adjunctive therapies often accelerate the entire healing process and promote improvement in spinal stability that could not be obtained otherwise.

The chiropractor, extensively trained in Physiological Therapeutics and aided by specialized equipment can supervise or administer the therapies right in the chiropractic office.

Some chiropractors do not provide physical therapy in their offices, but instead refer those patients needing the service to a physical therapist.

Chiropractic . . . and Acupuncture*

When newspaper reporters covering the visit to China by President Richard Nixon in 1972 began to write about the miracle of an ancient healing art, the concept immediately caught the American imagination. Suddenly, a new word was on everybody's lips: *acupuncture.*

According to the articles, instead of using chemical anesthetics during surgery, Chinese acupuncturists were somehow able to block the pain of surgery by painlessly inserting needles into the patient. Not only that, acupuncture relieved a wide variety of human ills, it was said, and had *worked reliably for hundreds of millions of persons through more than 4500 years of recorded history.*

With that kind of publicity, practically overnight, acupuncture was in great demand by Americans. Fortunately, hundreds of chiropractors throughout the nation already trained in acupuncture were ready to meet the demand.

---

*See "Scope of Practice" chapter.

Veterans of a "New Technique"

Chiropractors had been the first of the American healing professions to officially go to the Orient for the purpose of bringing acupuncture to the American people. Before that time, few American doctors of any kind knew anything about it. But several years before the Nixon visit, several thousand chiropractors had already begun to make use of acupuncture stimulation techniques including finger pressure, steel balls, heat, massage, blunt probes, electrical impulses and several kinds of needles. Chiropractors had been using the methods for so long they had even coined new terms such as "acutherapy," "acupoint," "acushock," "acu-exhaustion," and "acupressure," which are now standard terminology among acupuncturists.

The chiropractic profession's investigation into acupuncture officially began almost 20 years ago. In 1965, a small contingent of chiropractors traveled to Japan, Hong Kong and Taiwan to meet in a series of planned meetings with acupuncture delegates from those countries.

Those original meetings proved to be invaluable in breaking the ice. Then, in November 1967, several hundred Oriental acupuncture delegates met with a group of American chiropractors in Tokyo. All agreed that seminars for the training of chiropractors in the United States in acupuncture concepts and procedures should be instituted. A schedule for seminars to be held in the United States was arranged.

The first of these seminars was held in Kansas City, Missouri, in January, 1969. Dr. Leung Kok Yuen, Dr. Kunzo Nagayama, and Dr. Kenichiro Kon made the

41

long journey from the Orient and began a detailed explanation of the acupuncture principle and treatment procedure to nearly one thousand chiropractors from throughout the nation who attended the meeting. There, they began to learn Oriental healing wisdom nearly five thousand years old.

"Chi"

According to traditional acupuncture theory, the human body including the arms, legs, head, torso and internal organs is divided into zones called *meridians*. A special type of energy called *chi* circulates within and between the zones. A misdirection or other derangement of the energy flow results in disease or discomfort in the body. By stimulating specific zonal reflex points by needle, by hand or by other means, the acupuncturist can redirect and rebalance aberrations of the flow of *chi*.

The Chinese acupuncturist physicians of old discovered approximately 700 specific reflex points. In treating most conditions, several points must be stimulated simultaneously, sequentially or both, in order to redirect the healing energy into the area of disease or discomfort. This requires a great deal of training, knowledge and skill.

"Sister" Philosophies

From the beginning, the philosophy of acupuncture made sense to the chiropractors. After all, both disciplines, chiropractic and acupuncture, were concerned with normalizing energy systems in the body. Chiropractors normalize the *nerve* energy system of the body while acupuncturists normalize the *meridian* energy (chi) system of the body. It became obvious to the chiropractors attending those historic first meetings that despite the enormous cultural differences from which the two professions originated, chiropractic and acupuncture were "sister" philosophies.

During the next few years, ignoring the ridicule of acupuncture by medical doctors quoted in the press, acupuncture training seminars for chiropractors were held in major cities throughout the United States. And clinical trials and research programs to statistically validate the efficacy of acupuncture treatments were begun.

A Healing Combination

As a result of clinical experience, the interrelationship of acupuncture and chiropractic became very clear. It was observed that misaligned vertebrae affecting the nerve system brought on imbalance in the meridian system and vice versa. And, it was well-known that either chiropractic or acupuncture was capable of activating a flow of healing energy into the area of disease.

But it was seen that when acupuncture and chiropractic treatments were combined, the results were sometimes quicker and longer lasting.

From then on, chiropractic interest in acupuncture quickened. The first major textbook for training U.S. physicians in acupuncture had been published by chiropractors in 1968. A few years later the first certification training program in acupuncture for chiropractors was established by the New York Chiropractic College.

During the initial certification training, several thousand chiropractors studied traditional Oriental acupuncture in courses presented under the auspices of the various chiropractic colleges. Many State Boards of Examiners soon adopted the demanding criteria established by the college programs. Much of this spadework had either been accomplished or set in motion before the Nixon visit to China and the resulting publicity about acupuncture.

It was largely that attention which prompted the first positive interest in acupuncture of American medical physicians. Until then, with few exceptions, they had been highly critical of acupuncture even though a substantial number of medical doctors in Japan, England, France and Germany were utilizing acupuncture in their practices and were acclaiming its benefits.

American Awakening

Following the awakening of American medical physicans to the value of acupuncture, the chiropractic profession generously opened its acupuncture training seminars to dentists, veterinarians, medical and osteopathic physicians, permitting them to quickly develop their own expertise in acupuncture.

Chiropractic physicians were the first profession to have seen the enormous value of this ancient healing method.

Basing the initial amalgamation of chiropractic and acupuncture on the simple creed that the human body has the innate ability to cure its own ills, Oriental acupuncturists and American chiropractors leaped over language, technical, and other cultural barriers to meld the forty-five-century-old art of acupuncture with the modern methods of chiropractic.

Chiropractors are proud to have led the way in bringing the healing benefits of acupuncture to the American people.

Today, nearly all chiropractic colleges offer acupuncture courses in their graduate training programs and thousands of chiropractors utilize chiropractic *and* acupuncture to get sick people well.

Chiropractic . . .
and Nutrition

At first glance it may seem that nutrition and chiropractic have little in common. Nutrition has to do with proper nourishment of the body. Chiropractic has to do with proper nerve supply and function. However, these two disciplines work in tandem in the chiropractor's office, especially in diseases exhibiting nutritional deficiency.

Suprisingly, many chronic disease conditions arising from nutritional deficiency *do not respond to nutrition therapy alone.* But, when a combination of chiropractic treatments and a corrective nutritional regimen are followed, the results are often astounding. Here's why:

Each of the body's trillions of cells is a microscopic factory responsible for compounding chemicals essential for life and health. In all, thousands of different chemicals are manufactured within the body itself and delivered to other cells as needed.

In order to function as chemical factories, all the different kinds of cells, including the highly specialized cells of the nerves, require a balanced supply of raw materials: carbohydrates, fats, proteins, vitamins and minerals. These are the nutrients in food and food supplements.

When cells "run short" of certain nutrients, they are forced to slow down in their jobs of making certain chemicals and a sort of negative chain reaction begins, causing the body to slowly slide into chronic diseases.

Nutritional deficiencies are due to *either or both* of two factors:

(1) an inadequate or imbalanced intake of nutrients.
(2) the body's inability to assimilate or utilize the nutrients taken in.

Factor No. 1 might seem simple to solve by just eating a well-balanced diet. But, improper growing, harvesting, handling, shipping, storing, processing and preparing of food greatly diminishes its nutritional potency. So, a person may not be able to eat enough to correct nutritional deficiencies of long standing, or deficiencies caused by the side-effects of prescription drugs, street drugs, alcohol, smoking, surgical operations, emotional imbalance and stress and malnutrition itself.

When nutritional *intake* is a part of the problem in deficiency, a dietary regimen and probably a detailed food supplement program must be initiated to correct the problem. Most patients are unable to do this without expert help. The existing knowledge is enormous, expanding rapidly and bewildering to the untrained mind. Its complexity and ramifications exceed the understanding of most patients except those involved in nutrition professionally.

We can't expect effective dietary advice from more than a small percentage of medical practitioners, either. It's estimated that only about 30% of medical students receive even a smattering of specialized training in nutrition. To make up for a lack of specific courses in nutrition, medical schools gloss it over by teaching that a "well-balanced" diet will solve most nutritional deficiencies. Such a generalization may sound reassuring to patients, but it is scientifically untenable.

State of the Art Advice

Fortunately, to understand the importance of nutrition in restoring and maintaining health we can turn to the chiropractor for state-of-the-art nutritional advice.

Chiropractors have long enjoyed the reputation of being *the* experts in nutrition and nutritional counseling, *largely due to intensive study in college.* Since the chiropractor is the doctor concerned with natural health and maintenance of the body's natural immunity to disease, chiropractic colleges place strong emphasis on nutritional training.

Chiropractic license renewal programs require continued education, annually. Through these programs, chiropractic physicians have the opportunity for frequent updating in the latest clinical laboratory tests and procedures for evaluating the nutritional states of patients.

Also, through the American Chiropractic Association's Council on Nutrition, doctors of chiropractic can keep informed of new discoveries as they occur in the fast-paced world of nutrition. Most chiropractic journals publish regular updates on nutrition, too.

Altered Body Functions

But let's not forget that the appropriate intake of nutrition is only one factor in nutritional deficiency. The second factor in many cases is a diminished ability of the body to absorb, assimilate and utilize nutrients, even when intake is sufficient. Frequently, this inability is caused by altered nerve supply which alters functions of the body systems involved in digestion and assimilation.

When this happens, not only the other cells of the body but the nerve cells themselves can become undernourished. This condition impairs nerve functions in directing and controlling digestion and assimilation, which further starves the nerves and affects their function. It's a vicious circle diminishing the body's nutritional efficiency.

That's why nutritional counseling along with chiropractic treatments work wonders in restoring health.

It's an unbeatable combination, one you can't find anywhere else.

Chiropractic . . . and Psychology

Since mental and emotional stresses and problems can and often do affect physical health, patients should feel free to discuss such problems with the chiropractor.

Part of a chiropractor's pre-professional and professional education includes courses in psychology. Many chiropractors have undergraduate or graduate degrees in psychology.

Chiropractic studies in psychology courses cover current psychological theory and practice. Emphasis is placed on application of this knowledge to the care of the chiropractic patient.

Chiropractors receive training in the diagnosis of psychological disorders, behavior assessment, behavior therapy and psychotherapy.

While most chiropractors seldom do much formal counseling, all chiropractors are concerned with each patient's mental and emotional well-being.

If there is a need or a desire for intensive counseling, the chiropractic physician can refer the patient to appropriately qualified counselors or psychologists.

Chiropractic . . . and Acute vs. Chronic Diseases

There are two broad degrees of disease: acute and chronic. Doctors of chiropractic treat them both.

An *acute* disease usually requires immediate intervention because the disease is often rapidly on its way to becoming a crisis or has already entered a critical stage. Perhaps life or death is the issue of the moment.

A *chronic* disease usually has continued for a long time, perhaps coming and going in its symptom display, usually getting worse as time goes by.

Chronic disease has a bio-negative momentum. If that momentum is not stopped or reversed into a bio-positive momentum, the disease may become degenerative . . . even deadly.

High blood pressure is a typical example of a chronic disease that if untreated may cause a fatal stroke.

Although there is some flexibility in the dividing line between when an acute condition has become chronic, there is generally enough definition to decide upon the proper kind of treatment.

Some acute problems are emergency, life-threatening situations, requiring immediate intervention with powerful drugs or surgery. It is in this area of acute problems that the medical doctor's skills are most helpful. But less serious acute problems as well as the majority of chronic problems constitute the great bulk of the pains, complaints and miseries of the human race and in general respond well to chiropractic care.

Because chiropractors treat so many patients having chronic diseases, their D.C. degree is sometimes lovingly and humorously referred to as meaning "Doctor of Chronics." That's not surprising because their training, their experience and their wholeness philosophy are so well-suited to the treatment of chronic diseases and conditions.

The sensible approach to *any* disease condition is to utilize the most conservative intervention which will reverse the disease momentum.

Chiropractic . . . and Infectious Diseases*

Chiropractors treat infectious diseases and usually with excellent results.

In order to understand why and how drugless chiropractic treatments can affect infectious diseases, consider this:

Our world is loaded with microscopic organisms such as viruses, bacteria, spores, fungi, parasites, etc. —all commonly referred to as "germs" or "bugs."

Some are harmless. Some are essential to our well-being. Some are virulent and disease-related. Some of the latter are infectious and can be transmitted by direct contact or close proximity to the source.

Every time we go to a movie, sports event, or even the grocery store, wherever we come into contact with one or more persons, we increase the possibility of the introduction into our own bodies of all of the above organisms. Some of these organisms have the potential to produce disease. And it's important for everyone to understand that chiropractors are aware that "germs and viruses" *do* have their effect in *some* disease processes.

---

*See "Scope of Practice" chapter.

Indeed, the chiropractic viewpoint coincides with today's scientific viewpoint that many such disease-producers are already present in the body or the near-by environment most of the time. They are opportunistic, only waiting for a weakening in the host body so that they can then multiply and thereby cause a problem. Keep in mind that as long as the organisms are in small numbers and cannot multiply into colonies, they pose no immediate threat to human health.

Built-in Immunity

Most of us are born with a relatively strong auto-immune system which attacks and destroys most disease-producing micro-organisms, and during the process develops anti-bodies to be ready for the next onslaught of invaders.

Most infectious diseases have their own time span and are self-limiting. During the time span of the illness, the human body is creating anti-bodies which not only kill off the invading organisms, but often remain circulating in the bloodstream. This gives a long-term immunity and prevents recurrence of the disease. *This is a major benefit of naturally occurring anti-bodies over prescribed anti-biotics.*

However, if the auto-immune system is not functioning properly, the organisms can multiply and become overwhelming.

Occasionally, we hear of a child who was born with a *defective* auto-immune system who cannot go to the movies, to church or to any public gathering because, having no internal defense mechanism, the child becomes overwhelmed by the sheer volume of disease-producing organisms projected by a mass of people. Often, a child with this problem cannot have any human contact at all and has to live in a plastic bubble while waiting for a solution to the defect in the immune system.

The Struggle Within

Most of the time, the rest of us, because we possess a normal, healthy auto-immune system, resist all of the "bugs" being exchanged and transmitted through human contact, the atmosphere or other means. And we do it without even being aware of the struggle within.

The question, then, is not whether germs cause disease but, rather, what causes the body's auto-immune system to become so ineffective as to allow germs to take over?

Susceptibility to disease organisms is increased by vertebral misalignment, fatigue, exposure, malnutrition, environmental contaminants, toxins, poisons, certain drugs and mental and emotional strain.

Stress . . . and Distress

In fact, when the total stress levels of the body reach the *distress level*, the auto-immune system can become suppressed or overwhelmed. When that happens, the pathogenic (disease-producing) organisms, which are by nature opportunistic, can multiply at an unbelievable rate which in turn further overloads the auto-immune system. Then, we become victims of infectious disease.

Anything that lowers our vital resistance or suppresses the auto-immune system or breaks through any of the body's systems of defense can open the door to infectious diseases.

When the auto-immune system has become weakened, taking anti-biotics and other drugs can help to curb and control the invading organisms. But they cannot do the job totally on their own. The most powerful manufactured anti-biotics known are ineffective in the absence of a functioning auto-immune system. (Remember the child in the bubble).

Bringing Back Normal Function

Chiropractors do not treat these diseases directly, but, instead, treat them by restoring normal function to the nervous system which in turn directs and largely controls the functioning of the auto-immune system. The very presence of an infectious or contagious disease implies a reduced function and effectiveness of the patient's auto-immune system.

Chiropractors focus their efforts on restoring the normal potency of the patient's auto-immune system, permitting it to develop the phagocytes, anti-bodies and other defenses necessary to conquer the invading organisms and to restore health.

While anti-biotics do an excellent job of controlling infections, they are powerless to prevent them . . . and unless the underlying weakness in the auto-immune system is corrected, we may recover from an infectious disease (through anti-biotic therapy) only to remain highly susceptible to a recurrence or to other infections.

So that there's no misunderstanding, let it be known that chiropractors realize fully the benefits of anti-biotic therapy in infectious diseases. Some organisms are so virulent that they overwhelm even the healthiest auto-immune system. Some persons with a weak auto-immune system need help to cope.

But everyone should be mindful that such drugs can have dangerous side-effects and limitations for some people and therefore should be reserved for the most serious, critical cases.

Chiropractic . . . and Professional Education

The similarity between a medical and a chiropractic education is astonishing.

Both chiropractic and medical degrees require a minimum of six academic years to obtain. Applicants for chiropractic college must have completed at least two academic years (60 semester credit hours) of undergraduate credit leading to a baccalaureate degree at an accredited college or university. The chiropractic curriculum consists of four academic years of rigorous study and training in a chiropractic college. This makes a total of six academic years for the degree of Doctor of Chiropractic, (D.C.).

Medical schools also require a minimum of two years of pre-professional courses and an additional four years of medical courses for a total of six years to obtain the degree of Doctor of Medicine, (M.D.).

The majority of courses for either the D.C. or M.D. degree are essentially the same. However, certain of the chiropractic courses such as Chiropractic Spinal Analysis and Chiropractic Technique are absent in the medical curriculum. And, certain of the medical courses such as pharmacology and surgical procedures are absent in the chiropractic curriculum. But, either degree, D.C. or M.D., requires a minimum of six years.

Clinical Experience

Part of the training for either a chiropractor or a medical doctor is in clinical experience, sometimes called internship. In chiropractic colleges, the student usually interns in the college clinics. Generally, medical students intern in a hospital where they, too, learn the practical application of diagnosing and treating.

Also, each profession offers additional training for those doctors who wish to become specialists. The specialist training is termed "residency."

Although the length of the curriculum and the courses taught are essentially the same for chiropractic and medical physicians, the question arises: Are the two curriculums equal in quality? The question can best be answered by relating the now famous "basic science story."

Historic Test

More than forty years ago, the medical establishment (sharp-shooting at the chiropractic profession as usual) contended that the education of a chiropractor was inferior to a medical education. In an attempt to demonstrate medical superiority, the medical establishment successfully persuaded many state legislatures to pass "basic science" laws. These laws required chiropractors to pass the same basic science examinations for licensing as medical doctors.

The basic science examinations included such subjects as: anatomy, physiology, chemistry, bacteri-

59

ology, etc., the very subjects in which the medical establishment felt sure they would excel and thus expose the comparative inferiority of chiropractic education.

The result is history. Chiropractic students taking the same basic science exam, seated side by side with medical students in the examination room, *did just as well* as the medical students.

Each year since that time, chiropractors have repeatedly shown by such examinations that they are equally well-educated in all the basic health care sciences.

Additional Safeguards

Another safeguard that assures quality education in chiropractic colleges is the approval of a college by the Council on Chiropractic Education (CCE) which has its criteria approved by the United States Office of Education (USOE).

After the D.C. or M.D. degree is conferred, the doctors still face further examination before obtaining a license to practice in the state of their choice.

Both the chiropractic and medical professions have their own National Examining Boards where new graduates must pass examinations in *basic science* subjects as well as additional examinations in special subjects specifically applicable to each profession. Nearly every state accepts the test scores of the National Boards.

But, each state also requires that additional state examinations must be passed before a license is issued to either a chiropractor or a medical doctor.

On the next page is a selected list of courses taught in a typical chiropractic college.

Selected List of Courses Taught in a Typical Chiropractic College

Anatomy
Histology
Spinal Anatomy
Neuroanatomy: Brain,
  Spinal Cord, and
  Peripheral Nervous System
Human Genetics and
  Embryology
Axial and Upper
  Appendicular Anatomy
Abdominal and Lower
  Appendicular Anatomy
Normal Radiographic Anatomy
Physiology: Cellular-
          Neuromuscular
Physiology: Neuroendocrine
Physiology: Renal-Digestive
Physiology: Cardiovascular-
          Respiratory
Biochemistry
Toxicology
Nutrition
Cellular Pathology
Pathology of GI-GU Systems
Pathology of the Nervous
  System and Genetic Diseases
Pathology of the Cardiovascular
  and Respiratory Systems
Microbiology
Public Health, Hygiene, and
  Sanitation
Physical Diagnosis
Orthopedics
Clinical Laboratory Methods
Gastrointestinal and
  Genito-Urinary Diagnosis

Obstetrics
Psychology-Psychiatry
Infectious Diseases
Neurology
Dermatology-Syphilology
Eye, Ear, Nose, and Throat
Gynecology
Pediatrics
Geriatrics
Cardiovascular-Respiratory
  Diagnosis
Clinical Laboratory Diagnosis
Emergency Methods
X-Ray Physics and Technology
Roentgen Interpretation
Bone Pathology
X-Ray Pathology:
  Chest and Abdomen
Principles and Philosophy of
  Chiropractic
Fundamentals of
  Health Sciences
Chiropractic Spinal Analysis
Biomechanics
Chiropractic: Spine
  Adjustments
Chiropractic Technique
Jurisprudence
Chiropractic Clinical
  Principles
Research Methodology
Clinical Practicum
  (Public Clinic)
Physiotherapy
Kinesiology
Hospital Protocol

Chiropractic . . . and Pain

Pain in some part of the body is the main complaint of more than fifty percent of first-time chiropractic patients. The pain may be a headache, backache, shoulder ache, stomach ache or an ache any place. Something hurts somewhere. And many of these aching patients have been taking pain killers for years with no permanent relief. Some have even become addicted to the drugs without gaining permanent relief from pain.

Of course, none of us would choose to live in a world where pain medication was unavailable for intractable pain or incurable disease. And without question, anesthetics have their value and place.

But, the facts are that the majority of pain medications consumed in this country is not for intractable pain or disease. Instead, as the TV commercials inform us, more than one million Americans take Excedrin for headaches . . . *every day*. This TV statistic does not account for the other millions who take aspirin, Bufferin, Tylenol, Anacin, and so on. Nor are the other millions counted who take "temporary pain relievers" for sore throats, sinusitis, bursitis, neuritis, arthritis, muscle pain, upset stomach and a score of other ailments and discomforts.

Masking the Problem

Most people see little harm in this. But the chiropractic viewpoint is that if a person insists upon taking pain medication for "temporary relief," it should never be taken for anything more than a "temporary condition." Chiropractors know that pain killers do not reach or treat the underlying cause of the pain. They only mask or cover up the pain. Doing so often allows a minor problem to become major or an acute problem to become chronic.

Chiropractors, therefore, urge patients who find themselves repeatedly resorting to pain medication for recurring or chronic problems to be acutely conscious that the relief obtained is doing absolutely nothing to correct the underlying cause of the pain . . . but may, in fact, even allow the problem to become progressively worse and entrenched.

Much of chiropractic's reputation has been built upon its ability to relieve pain. Yet, its primary mission is to discover and *eliminate the underlying cause and source of the pain.*

Then, pain can go away and stay away.

Chiropractic . . . and Surgery

While chiropractors do not perform surgery,* they recognize the need and value of many surgical procedures and often refer patients for surgery.

But, they are also well aware that much unnecessary surgery is performed. Even the medical establishment itself is alarmed at the number of unnecessary surgical operations and is also concerned that surgeries do not always accomplish their purpose.

At best, any surgical procedure is dangerous, a form of benign violence as far as the body is concerned. Any thinking person would have to agree that if a conservative non-surgical procedure is known to have frequently worked in a specific condition, it should be tried first.

For nearly one hundred years, chiropractors have been correcting health problems, often after surgery has failed. It's obvious that in those instances, surgery could have been avoided by those patients going to the chiropractor first.

That's why chiropractors often say, "try chiropractic first, surgery last."

---

*In the state of Oregon, chiropractors are licensed to perform minor surgery.

Chiropractic . . . and Hospitals

In the past, with little exception, hospitals were of, by and for the medical profession—a profession which deliberately excluded chiropractic and chiropractors.

The self-serving aspect of this prejudice is being challenged everywhere. Many state legislatures have recently passed laws which allow chiropractors to utilize hospital facilities, to be a part of the hospital staff and to have access to hospital records at the request of their patients.

In states where such laws have not yet been passed, most chiropractors have an arrangement with a medical physician which permits a hospitalized patient to receive the benefit of some chiropractic attention.

No doubt in the near future all chiropractors will have access to hospital facilities and staff privileges.

Chiropractic . . . and Insurance

Virtually all plans and policies of most insurance companies include chiropractic coverage. In recent years, most states have instituted insurance equality laws which require insurance companies to pay chiropractors on an equal basis with all other primary health care providers including hospitals and other physicians. This includes the following:

> Medicare and Medicaid*
> State Welfare
> Personal Health Insurance
> Worker's Compensation
> Union Insurance
> Personal Injury
> Liability
> Automobile Med-Pay
> Automobile No-Fault

Specific questions about your insurance coverage in either the United States or Canada may be directed to any local chiropractor.

---

* Coverage varies according to the state in which the patient resides.

Chiropractic . . .
and Children

"As the twig is bent so grows the tree."

No one really knows how many millions of adults now living with serious health problems would be healthy today if their parents had only seen to it that they had received regular chiropractic check-ups as children.

A recent survey of chiropractic practices revealed that more than half of the adult patients exhibited a spinal distortion and faulty function directly related to one or both of the following:

(1) Injuries as a result of the birthing process, especially common in forceps delivery.
(2) Childhood accidents, mishaps or injuries.

Most of those childhood-related spinal conditions could have been corrected rather easily if they had been treated by a chiropractor in the early stages. Unfortunately, the parents were undoubtedly unaware of the need for chiropractic care. Probably they did not even recognize the signs that a problem existed.

Major Factors

Let's take a look at the main factors that cause damage to a child's structure and what can be done about it.

First, there's the birthing process itself. During birth, an infant's neck bones, pelvic bones and hip bones are commonly, though accidentally, dislocated or partially dislocated.

Then, there are just the pitfalls of growing up. A child's physical structure is constantly being "bent out of shape" as the child stumbles, falls and tumbles, slides and rolls while learning to walk or later while at play.

Fortunately, most of these childhood incidents have no lasting consequence. Due to the elasticity of the child's bones, ligaments and cartilages, misalignments caused by bumps, knocks and falls usually correct themselves almost immediately. But *some childhood misalignments do not correct themselves.* Then, the child grows with a twisted and distorted spine, pelvis and hip joint. Unless parents know what to look for, their untrained eyes are unlikely to detect the early signs indicating that "the twig has been bent."

One of the major structural factors chiropractors look for in little children is a twisted or misaligned pelvis caused at birth or by a bump or fall. All too frequently, a torsion (twisting misalignment) of the pelvis has the effect of making one leg functionally shorter than the other.

When this happens during a child's growth period, the resulting imbalance and difference in the amount of weight carried on each leg can *actually* cause a difference in the growth rate of the two legs so that one leg grows slower and thus shorter than the other.* Since the feet, legs and pelvis are the foundations for the structure of the spine, it is imperative that, if at all possible, the legs grow to the same length. Otherwise, the child may develop a weak spine subject to spinal curvature, scoliosis, disc degeneration and certain forms of arthritis.

Minor Misalignment . . . Serious Distortions

Even a minor misalignment can lead to serious spinal distortions and, in extreme cases, to advanced scoliosis, surgery, and years of wearing a brace . . . all because the child did not receive periodic chiropractic check-ups and have minor problems corrected while it was easy to do so.

To be sure that the spine is given its best opporunity to grow straight and tall, most chiropractors offer an every-six-month check-up service for children, *at no charge*, to detect any structural problems before they become serious. These twice-a-year check-ups start before the child begins to stand and continue through the eighth year, then at least once a year through age sixteen or seventeen. By that age, growth in the spinal bones is nearly completed and problems related to structural growth are unlikely to occur.

The Gift of Health

If a child's spine is neglected or abused and not

---

* Heuter-Volkman rule.

checked periodically during the growing years, the seeds of a lifetime of back trouble may have been sown. One of the greatest gifts a parent can give a child is regular chiropractic check-ups to insure that "the twig" grows up to become a physically sound healthy adult. Every parent should be aware of the early signs of spinal distortion that can often be detected through simple home tests.

Home Test for Pelvic Torsion in Children

This test should be given at least once a month between the twice-a-year chiropractic check-up or immediately after falls, accidents, mishaps, etc.

(1) Child lies face down across the bed, with legs far enough over edge so that feet and toes point toward the floor. Shoes on.

(2) Parent brings child's ankles together. By looking at heels of shoes, parent can observe if one leg appears shorter than the other.

(3) Any noticeable difference (1/16 inch or more) in leg length is a strong indication that one or more of the major pelvic bones has become misaligned, a serious finding, especially in growing children.

(4) If there is a noticeable difference, the child should be taken to a chiropractor for a professional evaluation. If treated in

the early stages, such problems are usually quickly, easily and inexpensively corrected painlessly. If left uncorrected, they can lead to a lifetime of spinal and other health problems.

Special Note

Research shows that even a slight difference in leg length during a child's growing years can slow the growth of the shorter leg causing it to become progressively shorter. For this reason, even a slight difference in leg length should be professionally evaluated and corrected to help prevent the development of scoliosis or other serious spinal conditions.

Early Warning Signs of Spinal Distortion in Children

Hips not level
One hip more prominent than the other
One shoulder more prominent than the other
Shoulders not level
Head carried tilted to one side
Head carried forward with chin thrust out
One arm hangs lower than the other

If any of the above warning signs of spinal distortion are visible in your child, a chiropractic check-up should be scheduled at once. Usually, such problems are easily corrected by chiropractic care while a child's body is still elastic and flexible.

Chiropractic . . .
and Sports Injuries

The athlete and the chiropractor share a common goal. The one thrives on adventure, excitement, and pushing to the limit of physical endurance. The other stands at the ready to put the injured athlete back together again. It's a perfect relationship.

The good old days are now. As high technology continues to replace the human as mule in the home and workplace, never before have Americans had so much time and energy left over after work to enjoy sports and recreational activities as right now, and never before have there been so many sports and recreation-related injuries. . .about 50 million per year. Some are serious. Most are minor. All involve an upset in the rhythm of the injured body's structure and function and most require some degree of attention or special correction.

The tremendous increase in volume of such play-time injuries is new. As recently as the 1930s and early 1940s, sports and recreational injuries were relatively rare. Most working people spent their waking hours working, not playing. Ten-hour work-days, six days a week, were common for men who were too worn down after work to do much more than eat supper, listen to the radio for awhile and go to bed early.

Women were worse off. Their days consisted of one menial household task after another. Children today find it hard to believe that just a few years ago women actually wrung out the wash by hand, hung it in a weak, winter sun and hoped the long johns would dry before they froze. Under such bleak conditions, common to most of the people, recreation was a never-never land. No wonder people used to say, "A man works from sun to sun but a woman's work is never done."

Counting Fireflies As Recreation

Even in summer active recreations were few. A typical pastime was sitting on the front porch in the evening, counting fireflies, just waiting for a "decent" time to go to bed...only to repeat the sameness of yesterday and today, tomorrow. Occasionally, a Sunday family picnic and softball game broke the heaviness of the monotonous routine.

There were plenty of professional sporting events and plenty of spectators, but the activity was confined largely to professional athletes and the rich. Most people got their daily exercise from a double ration of plain hard work.

The one bright spot in an otherwise austere existence was the innate, irrepressible nature of kids to play. They generated their own fun, games and activities with sandlot baseball, kick-can, hide-and-seek, cowboys and Indians and other inventiveness.

But most adults, until World War II, led rather prosaic lives.

Time for Play at Last

The end of the war marked a departure from the standard work ethic and the beginning of an acceptance of the maxim: "All work and no play makes Jack a dull boy." Advancing technology in the factory, office and home resulting in shorter work hours, more long weekends, extended vacations and earlier retirements suddenly gave every man, woman and child some extra time and energy to play. Today, more than four out of every five Americans exercise their bodies and refresh their minds in one or more of about six dozen major sports and recreations.

Play Creates Jobs

Although it seems contradictory at first, this enormous propensity for play is actually creating new jobs, occupations and careers in the burgeoning $25-billion-a-year sports and recreation industry. The more Americans play, it seems, the more jobs they create for themselves.

As leisure time becomes more abundant, many sports are being redesigned to accommodate more people. For example, it used to be that if you wanted to snow ski, first you had to climb the mountain on foot. Today, the skier is whisked to the summit in a chair lift or gondola and can ski down several times a day. Any winter weekend finds hundreds of thousands of skiers with special clothing and equipment on the nation's slopes. And hotels, inns and restaurants which cater to skiers are sprinkled throughout the mountain chains.

Water skiing is a good example of updated recreation. Man-made lakes and more powerful boat motors make it possible for about fifteen million people to water ski each year, creating an entire new industry. And about forty million people fish those lakes and the oceans.

Everybody's Doing It

There are millions of bowlers, campers and hunters. More than 100 million people swim for sport, and surfing is a popular and demanding sport.

Church and community basketball, softball and volleyball teams engage countless millions more. Youngsters in every city, town and hamlet are involved in Little League ball, while football and basketball are played in nearly every junior high, high school and college across the land. Then there are joggers, bicyclers, tennis players, thousands of racquetball and physical fitness centers, jazzercise, aerobic and break dancers. You name it! Even the handicapped—once banished to sedentary lives in a wheelchair—are enjoying the here and now of individual and team sports. Just about everyone is involved in the excitement of physical activity for the fun of it...even if it's only walking.

But People Do Get Hurt

Yet, the piper demands to be paid for this enjoyment. The speedy motion involved in sports exacts its toll. People get hurt in the movement of play. About one out of ten recreational injuries is obviously serious. A few result in death and some are crippling.

Most injuries, even minor ones, tend to produce some degree of derangement of one or more of the body's joints and the supporting structures (muscle, ligament, tendon, cartilage, fascia) are frequently overstretched or torn to some extent. Given prompt professional attention and proper rehabilitative care, the majority of the seriously injured can be back at work and play again, usually as fit as before.

Time Bomb Injuries

It's the so-called minor injury typically receiving little or no professional attention that so often ticks away like a time bomb, only to explode later as a "bad back," "trick knee," weak wrist or ankle, disabling arthritis or other health problems.

The traditional medical approach to the treatment of such injuries is substantially different from the chiropractic approach. Generally, medical doctors don't realize how serious some minor structural injuries can be. They are not trained to think of the body as a whole in the sense of the ankle being connected to the leg, the leg to the hip (and so on throughout the body's entire structure), and that injury in one area may cause a structural compensation in another, particularly when the spine becomes involved. The traditional medical viewpoint is oblivious to the obvious: the *apparent* site of a structural injury does not always comprise the full extent of the problem. Even minor sprains and strains of an ankle, knee or hip often throw the entire bony framework of the body off balance. This results in spinal and other problems that only chiropractors are likely to look for as a matter of course.

Traditional medical treatment for such injured joints is to immobilize the joint by splinting or taping it for a prolonged period of time. Then immobilization is followed by extensive physical therapy to overcome the deleterious effects of the prolonged immobilization. Little, if any, manual manipulation is prescribed or administered.

Timing Is Critical

Chiropractic training for the treatment of joint injuries is considerably different. The goal is to correct the derangement (dislocation, subluxation, fixation, misalignment) and to mobilize the injured part as soon as possible. The chiropractor is taught to recognize *if and when* the joint should be immobilized, when it should be realigned through manipulation, and when mobilization treatment should begin. The timing of mobilization is most critical to avoid the side effects of prolonged immobilization. When done at the proper time, mobilization helps prevent the shortening of muscles and ligaments and the formation of fibrous tissue, adhesions and contractures in and around the joint.

Experienced Chiropractors

With few exceptions, medical doctors get little or no training or experience in modern manipulative techniques. Lately, some have begun to see the wisdom of chiropractic in joint rehabilitation and sometimes recommend manipulation and mobilizing treatments by a chiropractor. While osteopaths and some physical therapists do manipulation, the chiropractor is generally much more experienced. Collectively, chiropractors give more than one million manipulations per day. Individually, they give hundreds of manipulations every week...a million or more in a practice lifetime. It is that tremendous volume of experience that makes the chiropractor the doctor of choice in most sports injuries not requiring surgery.

Also, frequent sports injury seminars sponsored throughout the country by chiropractic colleges, state and national associations and orthopedic and sports injury councils make available to all chiropractors the very latest expertise in the manipulation and rehabilitation of such injuries. It's no wonder the chiropractor enjoys the reputation for getting injured professional athletes back in the game quickly and safely.

Chiropractors Treat Pros

The treatment and recovery of injured, top-ranking athletes is one of chiropractic's brightest showcases. Through in-depth television and other media coverage of major sports events, sports heroes and sports injuries, the public frequently is made aware when yet another sports idol is back in the game due to chiropractic care...often after other methods have left the athlete still warming the bench. Many professional and college teams have a chiropractor on staff or on call to look after an entire spectrum of sports-related problems from simple sprains and strains to more serious problems resulting from intensive training and hard, competitive play.

But what about the rest of the active world, the husbands, wives and children who injure themselves just having a good time in some kind of sport or recreation? All too often the injury is just ignored. A day or two of work or school is missed; the pain goes away and the person resumes life again.

Spartan Approach

That Spartan, "suffer-it-through" approach is one way of dealing with an injury. It used to be the only way, but it never has worked very well because neglect so often leads to residual weaknesses and chronic problems. A neglected minor injury may eventually cause more trouble than a severe injury that has been well cared for.

Better Safe Than Sorry

Regardless of who is injured, be it weekend golfer, ho-hum fisherman, Little Leaguer, pro football player or Olympic star, sports and recreational injuries, even mild ones, should always have a chiropractic evaluation. There is no virtue in building and maintaining a healthy body through sports activity today, if a neglected injury causes a health problem tomorrow.

Chiropractic . . . and Ageing

Sometimes a person's spinal problems can remain dormant for years—unnoticed due to the elasticity of the body in youth—only to flare up as the body structures begin to age. Often, the cause began years ago: a congenital defect, deformity, anomaly or architectural deviation of the spine . . . or an unnoticed spinal or pelvic injury at birth . . . or an untreated childhood accident or injury.

In youth, our ligaments, muscles, cartilages and tendons are quite flexible and elastic. We have a good sense of balance and strength. Consequently, our bodies may cope with spinal and pelvic problems with little or no discomfort or loss of mobility until much later.

After the age of fifty or so, that youthful "give" and elasticity in the supporting structures of the spine begin to leave us . . . and as time goes by . . . we are likely to experience more and more health problems related to the spine and nerves.

Obviously, it's best to locate genetic and traumatic spinal problems as early in life as possible, treat them

with chiropractic care, and thus, avoid a lot of problems in later years.

But some of us who are getting older did not have—
or take—the opportunity for adequate chiropractic
care in our youth. Even if that's the case, we don't
have to "just learn to live with it." Many spinal problems in an older person require only a minor correction. Perhaps just a slight rebalancing of the spine or
merely taking the stress and torsion out of the pelvis
will bring comfort.

Because they've learned how much better it makes
them feel, millions of people over fifty go to the
chiropractor regularly for gentle, safe chiropractic
treatments.*

That way, they feel younger, much longer.

---

* Medicare includes chiropractic coverage.

Chiropractic . . . and Staying Well

When you acquire a substantial sum of money, would it be best to seek out an investment counselor to show you how to keep it intact? Or would you wait until you had a financial crisis before getting advice?

How about your lawn? Does it go to weeds before you spruce it up? Or do you take "preventive measures?"

Waiting until you *must* do something is always more costly than preventive measures. Most of us apply this "prevention principle" to everything of value in our lives—except our health.

The reason is obvious: we are conditioned to thinking in terms of killing a disease rather than maintaining a healthy, whole body . . . one that can nullify the negative effects of its environment.

When you're in a healthy state is the ideal time to have a chiropractic check-up and also review your nutritional status. If you don't have a chiropractor, what better time to get acquainted with one? And to let him get acquainted with your spine at its best rather than when it's on its worst behavior?

If you presently have a chiropractor, but only go when there's trouble, you're just asking for more trouble.

It's better to let your chiropractor help you maintain the integrity of your spine and nerves while you're in a health momentum.

Chiropractic . . . and Health as a Fun Trip

It's a grim life when you're on a disease trip, trying to keep just a step ahead of one symptom after another. But a great many people are on that trip and don't know there's another way to go.

In contrast to the dreariness of a disease trip, a health trip can be one of the greatest adventures life has to offer. And fortunately, the choice of which trip you take is only a matter of perspective, a matter of deciding whether you're trying to get rid of disease or obtain health.

The only "ticket" necessary to take the health trip is your understanding that health is a momentum toward integration of the structures and functions of your body . . . a momentum toward being a whole person rather than a fragmented person. Then, beyond that understanding, to have the most fun on the trip, you'll need a *desire* to become as whole as you possibly can.

If you decide to go on a health trip, before starting, you need to know one more thing: this is a *solitary* trip, not a group tour.

You're . . . You

The reason you have to go it alone is that no other human body is exactly like yours, neither on the outside, nor on the inside. Just compare your hands with someone else's hands. You'll never find a duplicate structure. There are no duplicate structures of your heart, lungs, spinal column or any other part, either. Similar, yes. Duplicate, no. No group advice or treatment is valid for you. Your health *needs* are individual and specific.

Also, your health and fitness *goals* are *individualistic*. For example, not everyone is interested in running the Boston Marathon, and not everyone could expect to attain the degree of health and fitness necessary to try. However, many people want to run that race and are fit enough to do it. There are some people, though, who would be delighted if they could just walk unaided to the market everyday.

Both your health *needs* and health *goals* are, undoubtedly, different than anyone else's. Your health trip, then, must be ticketed just for you by a doctor who understands your individuality and comprehends the wholeness concept . . . a doctor who understands where you want to go, who is realistic about your potential for getting there, and who will outline the easiest, safest and fastest route.

A doctor of chiropractic.

The very moment you decide to take a health trip instead of a disease trip, the fun begins. There's the exciting anticipation of the trip, soon followed by feelings of joy, pride and independence—exaltation, if you will—as you begin to realize that your very own body is making itself whole again.

Chiropractic . . . and Its Limits

Q. Is chiropractic a cure-all?

A. Absolutely not. Yet, the limits of what chiropractic treatments can achieve are not yet fully known. Here's why:

Vertebral misalignments and the resulting nerve impingements *interfere* with the normal functions of the nervous system and thereby diminish the body's curative powers. *The chiropractor by correcting the vertebral misalignment thereby re-establishes nerve function and normalizes the body's curative powers.*

Once normalized, that power is awesome, but like gravity, goes unnoticed most of the time. Its tremendous significance is lost to our consciousness.

Small Demonstration of Great Power

For example, we take for granted the healing of wounds, cuts and lacerations. We seem unmindful of the body's ability in those instances to actually grow new flesh and skin in repairing itself. Yet, these everyday demonstrations are only one small aspect of the body's power to heal itself.

Perhaps because we can't see what is happening, we fail to realize that the same power that heals wounds on the *outside* of the body, heals functional and organic diseases on the *inside* of the body.

Scientists recognize the existence of this power, but so far, no one has documented its limits in affecting disease conditions. Since chiropractic focuses on this curative power, the parameters of chiropractic are still unknown.

We do know that the scope of chiropractic is broad, as broad as the nervous system which affects every tissue and every cell to some degree. Because chiropractors work chiefly with the spine and nerves, most people see them as the doctor of choice for back pain, and back problems.

The Whole Person

But many people are unaware that doctors of chiropractic treat the whole person for a long list of functional and organic diseases and conditions in all parts of the body. As a result of chiropractic research and the ongoing development of new technologies in diagnosis and treatment, the list of treatable conditions continues to grow.

Following is only a partial list of conditions for which chiropractic has an excellent treatment record.

This list is not intended to be exhaustive. There are hundreds of other conditions, syndromes and symptoms which frequently respond to chiropractic care.

When chiropractic is combined with acupuncture and nutritional counseling, the number of treatable conditions grows to an estimated four hundred or more.

Some of the Conditions Treatable by Chiropractors*

Allergies

Ankle Swelling

Arm and Shoulder Pain

Arthritis

Asthma

Back Pain—Backache—Low Back Pain

Bed Wetting (Enuresis)

Blood Pressure—High and Low

Bronchial Conditions

Bursitis

Chest Pains

Circulation, Poor

Colitis

Colon, Spastic

Constipation

Cough, Chronic

Diarrhea

Disc Problems

Diverticulitis

Dizziness (Vertigo)

Ear and Eye Problems

Emphysema

Fatigue, Chronic

Feet, Cold

Feminine Problems

Gall Bladder Disorders

Gas

Glandular Troubles

Hay Fever

Headaches

Headaches, Migraine

Heart, Fast or "Nervous"

Hemorrhoids

Hiccoughs

Impotence

Indigestion

Insomnia

Joint Pain

Kidney Problems

Knee Pains

Leg Cramps, Tingling and Numbness

Liver Problems

Neck, Stiff

Nervousness

Neuralgia

Pleurisy

Prostate Trouble

Rectal Itching

Rheumatism

Sciatica

Shingles

Shoulder Pain

Sinus Trouble

Sports Injuries

Stomach Problems

Throat, Sore

Thyroid Conditions

Ulcers, Stomach

Whiplash

*See "Scope of Practice" chapter.

Chiropractic . . .
and Scope of Practice

Each state reserves for itself the right to license all health care providers including doctors of chiropractic, medicine, osteopathy, optometry, dentistry, podiatry and psychology and to determine the scope of practice of each . . . that is, what each professional may or may not do in that particular state.

The scope of chiropractic practice varies from state to state because some state laws have not kept up with the progress in technological developments that are already included in chiropractic college curriculums, and therefore a part of chiropractic expertise.

For example a few states still restrict, in part or in whole, chiropractors from utilizing acupuncture, some physical therapy modalities, and limit the conditions chiropractors may legally treat.

Reasons for these variations in state laws are nearly lost in antiquity. When chiropractic began nearly one hundred years ago, many of the treatment modalities including acupuncture and modern physical therapies were either unknown or untaught and therefore not included in the state laws defining the scope of chiropractic.

Today, more and more, chiropractic scope-of-practice statutes are being updated to reflect the new discoveries and technological advances already being taught in chiropractic colleges.

Chiropractic . . . and the Chiropractic Career

Early in their lives many of today's chiropractors sensed the unique satisfaction of a career centered on relieving the pain and misery of seemingly desperate disease situations.

Others, later in their lives—even after success in another career—changed careers by going back to college for a chiropractic degree so they could help the sick. It is becoming common for people with Bachelor, Master, even Ph.D. degrees in totally different disciplines to become chiropractors. Some of these people made their decision after having had a personal "miracle" experience with chiropractic or after watching a sick friend or relative become whole again—literally—at the hands of a chiropractor.

And more and more sons *and daughters* of chiropractors are deciding it would be great to follow in dad's and grandfather's footsteps. They have grown up immersed in the wonder of chiropractic and have admired their parents' dedication to getting sick people well.

They want to be a part of that tradition.

But chiropractic is not a closed corporation. You don't have to already *be* part of the chiropractic family to *become* part of the family. Nor do you need a personal chiropractic experience.

To become a chiropractor you need only a good mind, a dedication to hard work, and a passion for helping your fellow man.

The special rewards of this special career include financial security as well as the knowledge that people really need your skills and talents.

Following is a list of chiropractic colleges in this country and abroad:

Chiropractic Colleges

CLEVELAND
CHIROPRACTIC COLLEGE
6401 Rockhill Rd.
Kansas City, MO 64131

CLEVELAND
CHIROPRACTIC COLLEGE
590 N. Vermont Ave.
Los Angeles, CA 90004

LIFE CHIROPRACTIC
COLLEGE
1269 Barclay Circle
Marietta, GA 30062

LIFE CHIROPRACTIC
COLLEGE–WEST
2005 Via Barrett, P.O. Box 367
San Lorenzo, CA 94580

LOGAN COLLEGE OF
CHIROPRACTIC
1851 Schoettler Rd., Box 100
Chesterfield, MO 63017

LOS ANGELES COLLEGE
OF CHIROPRACTIC
16200 E. Amber Valley Dr.,
Box 1166
Whittier, CA 90609

NATIONAL COLLEGE OF
CHIROPRACTIC
200 E. Roosevelt Rd.
Lombard, IL 60148

NEW YORK
CHIROPRACTIC COLLEGE
P.O. Box 167
Glen Head, NY 11545

NORTHWESTERN
COLLEGE OF
CHIROPRACTIC
1834 S. Mississippi River Blvd.
St. Paul, MN 55116

PALMER COLLEGE OF
CHIROPRACTIC
1000 Brady St.
Davenport, IA 52803

Chiropractic Colleges *(continued)*

PALMER COLLEGE OF
CHIROPRACTIC–WEST
1095 Dunford Way
Sunnyvale, CA 94087

PARKER COLLEGE OF
CHIROPRACTIC
300 E. Irving Blvd.
Irving, TX 75060

PASADENA COLLEGE OF
CHIROPRACTIC
1505 N. Marengo Ave.
Pasadena, CA 91103

PENNSYLVANIA INSTITUTE
OF STRAIGHT
CHIROPRACTIC
P.O. Box 849
Levittown, PA 19058

SHERMAN COLLEGE OF
STRAIGHT CHIROPRACTIC
P.O. Box 1452
Spartanburg, SC 29304

TEXAS CHIROPRACTIC
COLLEGE
5912 Spencer Hwy.
Pasadena, TX 77505

WESTERN STATES
CHIROPRACTIC COLLEGE
2900 N.E. 132nd Ave.
Portland, OR 97230

Australia
PHILIPS INSTITUTE OF
TECHNOLOGY
International College of
Chiropractic
P.O. Box 96
Bundoora, Victoria 3083,
Australia

SYDNEY COLLEGE OF
CHIROPRACTIC, LTD.
7 Esplanade
P.O. Box 42
Ashfield 2131, Australia

Canada
CANADIAN MEMORIAL
CHIROPRACTIC COLLEGE
1900 Bayview Ave.
Toronto, Ontario, Canada
M4G 3E6

England
ANGLO-EUROPEAN
COLLEGE OF
CHIROPRACTIC
13-15 Parkwood Road
Boscombe, Bournemouth,
Dorset, England BH52DF

France
INSTITUT FRANCAIS
DE CHIROPRACTIC
92 Bis Ave du General Leclerc
F95390 Saint Prix, France

Chiropractic . . . and The Future

"The doctor of the future will give no medicine but will interest his patients in the care of the human frame, in diet, and in the cause and prevention of disease."
—Thomas A. Edison

Chiropractic's turbulent past and dynamic present speak to us in no uncertain terms about its future. Just ninety years ago there was only one chiropractor, Dr. Daniel David Palmer. Today there are more than 32,000 licensed chiropractors world-wide, more than 25,000 practicing in all of the fifty United States. That's about one chiropractor to serve every ten thousand Americans—in comparison to one medical doctor for every six hundred citizens.

Clearly, more chiropractors are needed *now*.

The demand today for chiropractors and chiropractic treatments is unprecedented. The average number of patient visits per week per medical physician stands at 107. But, the average number of patient visits per week per chiropractor is almost the same and increasing steadily, an increase partially due to chiropractic's having broadened into acupuncture, reflex therapy and nutrition.

The Switch to Chiropractic
Every day more and more enlightened people shake

off the awkward yoke of total dependancy on medicine and drugs as they switch to chiropractic's modern health methods and concepts.

In addition, the passage of insurance equality laws guaranteeing even-handed payment of insurance claims also can be expected to dramatically increase the number of chiropractic patients.

But that's not all. Further increases in patient visits can be expected since some states now require the opening of public-funded hospitals to chiropractors. It is anticipated that chiropractors will have wide-open access to all hospitals in the near future.

Also, chiropractors are in the forefront of research and treatment in many of the new technologies such as laser bio-stimulation, electrical bio-stimulation, electro-magnetic fields, vibration therapy and color therapy. These new methods are well within the traditional domain and scope of chiropractic practice (manipulation supplemented with adjunctive, non-surgical, drugless methods) and may soon replace many chemical and drug treatments.

This outreach by chiropractors who are open-minded to new, non-invasive health care methods, and their enthusiastic acceptance by patients have been a part of chiropractic's validation process, a validation that has occurred rapidly over a span of only about three generations.

Burning Question

But now that the validation of chiropractic has been achieved, there remains one burning question: will there be enough chiropractors next year . . . and the next . . . and the next to fulfill the needs and wants of the people?

Certainly, chiropractic educators are working on the solution. To help meet the ever-increasing demand for more chiropractors, an average of one new chiropractic college has been opened each year for the past several years. This has doubled the number of colleges and students compared to just a few years ago. Also, several existing colleges are expanding their facilities to accommodate up to twice as many students as are currently enrolled.

But the education of the chiropractor takes a minimum of four academic years of intensive chiropractic college study and training. This is a time barrier that cannot be jumped over, rushed or compressed. At the present time, about 10,000 chiropractic students are enrolled and about 2,500 graduate each year. At that rate, there will still be less than 50,000 chiropractors at the end of this decade.

This will not be enough chiropractors. The demand is already beginning to overtake the supply.

Self Supporting

The growth of chiropractic educational facilities has always been curtailed due to discriminatory government policies which have funded medical schools and hospitals—but not chiropractic colleges. This has left the development of chiropractic colleges dependent almost entirely upon the contributions and donations of individual chiropractors.

So far, chiropractors themselves have come forward with the mental and financial capital necessary to found colleges, and make available a quality education to qualified men and women seeking a career in chiropractic. But with the increasing demand for chiropractors now and the immediate future, the availability of enough private capital to meet the educational demand could be a problem.

So, we still have the same question: will there be enough chiropractic college classrooms and other educational facilities to educate enough new doctors to meet the accelerating demand for chiropractic services? That is *the* question, and the future health of millions of Americans hangs on its answer.

Strong Leadership

When we examine our chiropractic leadership, we see that, happily, the answer is yes. Chiropractic leadership has never been stronger than it is today; it's getting stronger as more and more forward-looking men and women come into the profession.

With the quality of leadership available, the challenges of the future, somewhat different from those of the past, will be met and chiropractic will continue to fulfill its destiny.

And of one other constant we can be sure: chiropractors are dedicated to the integrated structure and function of the *whole* person. Nothing in the future will change that.

Chiropractic . . . and Exercise

Everyone agrees that exercise is essential to good health, yet there is often disagreement about what kind of exercise and how much exercise are necessary to achieve and maintain a reasonable level of physical fitness . . . a degree of fitness that allows you to do most of the things you want to do when you want to do them without undue pain or fatigue.

Most persons engaged in hard, manual labor or strenuous sports activities are sure they are getting plenty of exercise . . . and perhaps they are. Still, the question each person must answer is: *am I adequately exercising all of my muscles that need exercise?*

Probably not. Each of the body's muscles requires frequent use (exercise) in order to attain and maintain strength, balance, coordination and endurance. Insufficient exercise (use) of any one of them results in weakness and flabbiness of that particular muscle.

Joints Must Move

But there is more to fitness than strong and supple muscles. The body's supporting structures need exercise, too, and they get it when muscles are used. Muscles move the body's parts by moving its joints. When joints move, the supporting structures including ligaments, tendons, cartilages, membranes, capsules get the exercise vital to their good health.

To keep supporting structures strong, yet flexible and elastic, and to prevent the formation of adhesions, contractures and restricted range of motion, joints must be moved through their full range of motion each day. Since many occupations and sports activities fail to meet this requirement, hard work or strenuous exercise do not necessarily insure adequate exercise of all the muscles or complete range of motion of all the joints and supporting structures. Primary indicators of improper or inadequate physical activity include pain, weakness, stiffness and chronic tiredness.

"Canned" Exercise May Be Harmful

While there are numerous "canned" exercise and fitness programs of one kind or another always being marketed via fitness centers, books and videotapes, these generalized programs usually fail to consider that the intended customer may have some physical impairment, disability or health problem. They presume that the customer is fit enough to undergo the program.

Because generalized fitness programs can be harmful, even dangerous, for persons with a history of neck, back, hip, arm or shoulder problems, it is vital that evaluation of the individual's needs and limitations be made . . . preferably by a chiropractor . . . before starting any exercise or fitness program.

Chiropractors are extensively educated and trained in exercise physiology and a substantial portion of chiropractic practice involves treatment and rehabilitation for sports injuries, industrial injuries, auto accidents and other neuro-musculo-skeletal conditions. Combining chiropractic treatments and specific exercises is often the best method to get rid of back and neck problems and reduce the likelihood of recurrence.

Chiropractic and Exercise

Chiropractic treatments (called adjustments) realign the vertebrae to their proper position, thus freeing pinched or irritated nerves resulting from vertebral misalignments.

Specific exercises strengthen weak muscles, thus allowing the spine to attain and maintain its proper balance, flexibility, extensibility and stability. In turn, *this makes for longer-lasting effectiveness of the chiropractic treatments.* Until weak muscles are strengthened, the back tends to be unstable and subject to muscle spasms, vertebral subluxations, disc degeneration, pinched nerves, pain and other problems.

Strong Abdominal Muscles Vital

Strange as it may seem, weak abdominal muscles are more frequently a cause of low back pain than weak back muscles. The spine is supported from the back by back muscles. It is supported from the front by neck muscles in the neck area, the rib cage in the chest area and abdominal muscles in the lower spine area. If good spinal health is desired, muscles of the abdominal wall must be strong enough to compress the innards of the body snugly against the spinal column. In this way strong abdominal muscles shore up the lower spine holding it upright from the front.

In addition, a constant, subtle interplay of "give-

and-take" between the back muscles, hip muscles and abdominal muscles helps keep the spine balanced when it is erect. Obviously, if the back, hip or abdominal muscles are weak, the resulting muscular imbalance leads to instability of the spine and inevitably to back pain and problems. Good spinal health demands that both back muscles and abdominal muscles be reasonably strong and balanced.

Sitting Creates Problems

Weakened abdominal muscles are quite common. They tend to occur most often in those persons whose occupations or life-styles require a great deal of sitting. The sitting (flexed) posture sustained for long periods of time at a desk, typewriter, TV, computer console, automobile, truck, etc.—without sufficient offsetting exercise or physical activity—creates an imbalance between the opposing back muscles and abdominal muscles.

For that reason, the correction of many acute and chronic back problems requires strengthening exercises of both the back muscles and abdominal muscles to bring them into balance.

Chiropractic Evaluation Needed

The exercises in this chapter are suitable as an exercise and fitness program for persons who are in good health and without physical impairment or disability.

Some of the exercises shown may not be appropriate for certain individuals with physical disabilities or during certain phases of corrective and rehabilitative care. Any exercise program for such persons should be closely monitored and the patient's progress evaluated during the rehabilitation program. No exercise program should be started by a person with health problems or a history of neck, back or joint problems until the person's condition, needs and level of fitness have been evaluated by a chiropractor.

Flexion, Extension, Stretching, Strengthening and Rehabilitation Exercises

Any of the depicted exercises may, at times, be prescribed for the correction or rehabilitation of specific spinal disorders. However, the exercises do not encompass the entire range of available corrective and rehabilitative exercises. In some instances, other exercises may be recommended by the chiropractor.

Persons with back and neck problems should not attempt these exercises without getting specific recommendations from a chiropractor.

Doctor's Guidelines and Recommendations

_____

_____

_____

_____

_____

_____

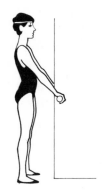

THE DOORKNOB STRETCH

A. Center self before open door, feet comfortably apart 6–8 inches from door. Grasp door handles.

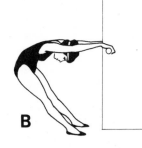

B. Lower buttocks as far as possible keeping arms and legs straight. Slowly count to four, then pull self to original upright position.
Begin with two sets. Progress to 6.

Doctor's Recommendations:

_____

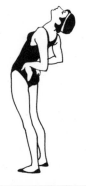

STANDING BACK STRETCH

Stand erect. Place hands as shown. Bend backwards to produce a gentle stretch. Hold to count of 3. Return to start. Begin with 3 sets. Progress to 10.

Doctor's Recommendations:

_____

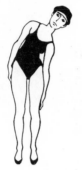

TORSO SIDE BENDS

Stand erect. Bend torso sideways from waist as far as is necessary to produce a gentle stretch. Hold for a count of 2. Repeat in opposite direction. Begin with 3 sets. Progress to 10.

Doctor's Recommendations:

_____

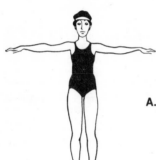

TORSO TWIST

A. Assume position shown.

A

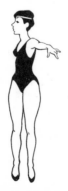

B. Slowly rotate torso to produce a gentle stretch. Then rotate in opposite direction.
Begin with 3 sets. Progress to 10.

Doctor's Recommendations:

_____

_____

B

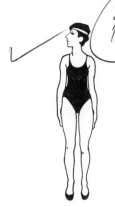

(handwritten: 2x day 10/14)

NECK ROTATION

Stand. Face straight ahead. Slowly rotate head and face to one side to produce a gentle stretch. Hold for count of 2. Return to start. Repeat in opposite direction. Begin with 3 sets. Progress to 10.

Doctor's Recommendations:

_____

_____

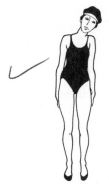

NECK BENDS

Lateral Bend

Slowly bend neck sideways to produce a gentle stretch. Hold for count of 2. Return to start. Then bend neck to opposite side. Hold for count of 2. Return to start. Begin with 3 sets. Progress to 10.

Doctor's Recommendations:

_____

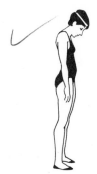

NECK BENDS

Forward Bend

Slowly bend neck forward to produce a gentle stretch. Hold for count of 2. Return to start. Begin with 3 sets. Progress to 10.

Doctor's Recommendations:

_____

_____

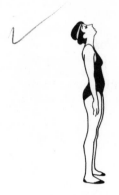

NECK BENDS

Backward Bend

Slowly bend neck backward to produce a gentle stretch. Hold for count of 2. Return to start. Begin with 3 sets. Progress to 10.

Doctor's Recommendations:

_____

_____

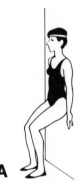

WALL SQUAT

A. Stand the length of your foot from the wall. Slide down wall until thighs are at angle shown. Hold until a mild strain is felt. (In beginning may be only a few seconds). Return to start position. Begin with 3 sets. Progress to 10. As the legs get stronger Exercise B may be attempted.

Doctor's Recommendations:

_____

_____

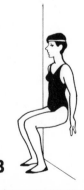

B. Same as Exercise A except that thighs are at angle shown.

Doctor's Recommendations:

_____

_____

1st 3 - 2x day
10 Repet φ each

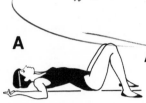

PELVIC TILT

A. Lie on your back, knees up. Rock pelvis by arching lower back as far as possible. Hold to count of ten.

B

B. Then rock pelvis in the opposite direction by flattening lower back against floor. Hold to count of ten. Begin with 3 sets. Progress to 10.

Doctor's Recommendations:

_____

_____

NOTE: Can also be done in standing position with knees slightly bent. Back against wall.

KNEE TO FOREHEAD

Lie on your back with knees up, as in Figure B of PELVIC TILT (above).

Pull one knee toward the head and raise the head toward the knee to produce a gentle stretch. Alternate right and left leg. Begin with 3 sets. Progress to 10.

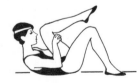

Doctor's Recommendations:

_____

BOTH KNEES TO FOREHEAD

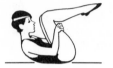

Using both knees, follow directions for ONE KNEE TO FOREHEAD.

Doctor's Recommendations:

_____

_____

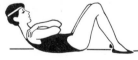

2 x day
work up to 20 left

CURL UPS

Lie on back with knees up, arms outstretched. Raise head and shoulders from the floor. Return to starting position. Begin with 3 sets. Progress to 20. Then progress to ADVANCED CURL UPS, A and B.

Doctor's Recommendations:

_____

_____

ADVANCED CURL UPS—A

Arms across chest. Follow CURL UP directions.

Doctor's Recommendations:

_____

_____

ADVANCED CURL UPS—B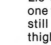

Hands clasped behind neck. Follow CURL UP directions.

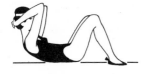

Doctor's Recommendations:

_____

_____

HAMSTRING STRETCH

Lie on back, knees up. Raise one thigh straight up with knee still bent. Clasp hands behind thigh. Gradually straighten leg as far as possible to produce a gentle stretch. Alternate legs. Begin with 3 sets. Progress to 10.

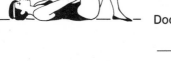

Doctor's Recommendations:

_____

HIP ABDUCTION

Lie on side as shown. Raise leg as far as you can to produce a gentle stretch. Hold for count of 2. Return to start. Begin with 3 sets. Progress to 10. Then alternate legs.

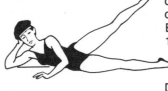

Doctor's Recommendations:

_____

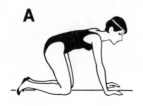

THE TORSO STRETCH

A. Assume crawl position as shown.

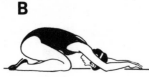

B. Then assume position as shown. Forehead against floor, arms extended. Hold to count of four. Return to crawl position. Begin with 3 sets. Progress to 10.

Doctor's Recommendations:

_____

_____

PRESS UPS

A. Assume position shown. Toes on floor.

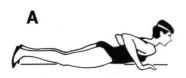

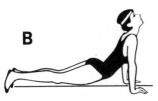

B. Straighten arms to press up into position shown. Hold for count of 2. Return to start. Begin with 3 sets. Progress to 10.

Doctor's Recommendations:

_____

_____

TORSO AND LEG LIFT

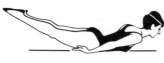

Lie face down. Hands at side. Raise head, chest and legs at same time by arching lower back. Hold to count of 10 if you can. Return to start position. Begin with 3 sets. Progress to 10.

Doctor's Recommendations:

_____

_____

DONKEY KICKS

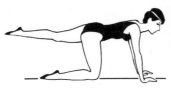

Start in crawl position. Raise one leg by extending it straight. Hold for count of 3. Return to start position. Alternate legs. Begin with 3 sets. Progress to 10.

Doctor's Recommendations:

_____

_____

A

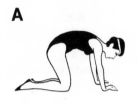

SWINGING BRIDGE

A. Assume crawl position as shown.

B

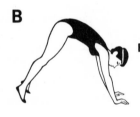

B. Raise self to bridge position. Hold for count of 2.

C

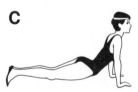

C. Swing through to press up position by sliding legs backward. Hold to count of 2. Return to position B. Then go back to position C. Return to start. Begin with 1 set. Progress to 4.

Doctor's Recommendations:

_____

_____

A

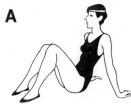

REVERSE SWINGING BRIDGE

A. Assume position shown.

B

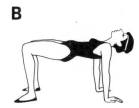

B. Then assume position B. Hold for count of 2.

C. Then swing through to Position C. Hold for count of 2. Swing back to position B. Hold for count of 2. Then swing back to Position C. Hold for count of 2. Return to position A. Begin with 1 set. Progress to 4.

C

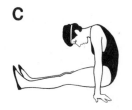

Doctor's Recommendations:

_____

_____